I0435667

The Beginners Guide to Medicinal Plants

BY LINDSEY P

Everything You Need to Know About the Healing Properties of Plants & Herbs, How to Grow and Harvest Them

2nd Edition

Table Of Contents

Introduction

I want to thank you and congratulate you for purchasing the book, *"The Beginners Guide to Medicinal Plants"*.

This book contains proven steps and strategies on how to successfully grow medicinal plants and herbs right at the very comfort of your own home.

Featured in this book are some of the most common mistakes when putting up a medicinal garden at home and how to avoid committing such mistakes. Also featured in this book are some of the best types of medicinal plants to grow at home.

Thanks again for purchasing this book, I hope you enjoy it!

Chapter 1: Guide to Growing a Medicinal Herb Garden

Growing medicinal plants and herbs indoor is a popular hobby for a lot of gardeners. One of the greatest reasons to plant medicinal plants indoor is to have a ready supply of these beneficial herbs. These herbs are those that you commonly snip into your sauces and soups. They can also be used to soothe an itchy rash or cough. Growing medicinal herbs may not sound to be very appealing, however you can benefit from growing these plants that can provide instant relief for many illnesses that can happen anytime of the day.

It would also be wonderful to be able to cut a sprig of thyme while boiling water and prepare a fresh cup of thyme tea that is fragrant and vibrant. Since it is fresh, you'll sure it is effective since it's fresh.

So what kind of medicinal plants should you grow? The next chapter of this book features a list of different herbs and medicinal plants that you can grow at home. The list is just a good starting point for easy to find and easy to grow herbs. The same plants that you can use in cooking daily may also be used as teas, salves, washes and tinctures. You can also make cough syrup and cough drops with the very same herbal plants that you grow in the comforts of your own home.

No matter how you thoroughly care for your medicinal plants, in the long run, they will have to be replaced. If this should happen during the colder days, you will have to take into account the growing time, before they will be big enough for harvest. Commonly, this will take about 4 to 6 weeks. You can make use of these herbs not only for cooking but for medicinal purposes as well.

What problems can you possibly encounter while growing medicinal plants and herbs in your home garden? While herbs typically suffer from much less issues that flowers and vegetables do, there are a few things that should be looked out for. Plants grown in your home garden may also encounter some basic problems such as molds or mildew problems, insect damage and most of all, fertilizer issues. To remedy these problems, you must know the following guidelines:

1. Home Garden Temperature

   While most of us think our homes as a temperate area would be ideal for growing plants, this is not always the case.

   A plant requires light in order to make food, a process which we know as photosynthesis. While plants are very adaptable, they grow best within a 70 to 75 degree range. A plant utilizes more energy when the temperature is warm than when it is cold. Plants can adapt to a cooler room, for instance, with an air conditioner. The plants will begin the process of photosynthesis with the increase in temperature and there will be no sunlight to produce food. When this happens, the plants will not most likely to thrive and will probably die.

   So what is the best temperature for growing medicinal herbs?

   Plants grow best when there is at least a 10 degree fall in temperature during the night. During the summer, the temperature tends to get high and stay high. Plants get stressed and become highly susceptible to diseases. They grow less and can drop leaves, weaken and die, despite sufficient watering. If you are growing herbs indoors, it would be a good idea to grow them around a room based on available temperature zones. Save a lot of money and be stress-free by working on with what you already have instead of trying to make big modifications that work against the natural rhythm of your home environment.

2. Home Garden Fertilizer

Once you have already decided on which type of herbs that you will grow in your home garden, you will now have to choose the most suitable fertilizer for them. Not all fertilizers are created the same. While most have advertising claims, these fertilizers may be overused enough to damage your medicinal herbs grown at home.

What kinds of fertilizers can be used at home? There are a lot of fertilizer types that will work for your medicinal herb garden at home. For indoor plants, you can try using a variety that can be dissolved in water (water-soluble). This particular type of fertilizer may come in packaged granular form that you measure and dissolve in water prior to application. It may also come in the form of a fish emulsion, which is a concentrated variety and is combined with water before application.

Regardless on the type of fertilizer that you choose to use, you must apply it at one quarter of the packaging's recommended amount. Apply this light mixture once every week. For a more effective application, make sure to water your plants thoroughly and then apply the prepared fertilizer solution. This technique will allow for better absorption by the plant.

More importantly, make sure that you do a monthly flushing of your medicinal plants. This can be done by placing the plant in a sink and water entirely, allowing the excess water to draw off. Once the dripping stops, water completely once again. This technique will get rid of any salts that may have accumulated in the plant's soil.

3. The Location of Your Garden Matters

One important thing that you must think about is the location of their home garden. Some people may have a traditional yard garden in mind when they think about planting herbs. If you have enough space in your backyard, then this gardening method will work quite well for you. However, if you lack gardening space then you will have to employ some ingenuity.

This is where alternative gardening methods come in. Some people plan their gardens near window sills inside pots. Some people prefer to plant their herbs in containers and move the plants around as needed. Remember that some herbs require more sunlight than others. A mobile container herb garden may be a better option for people who live in urban settings where access to large plots isn't always possible.

Container gardening entails less work since you'll be working on less space. Of course, that also means you will only have a smaller yield, which is a bit of a downside in case you're growing medicinal herbs for more people. However, a window sill garden isn't as prone to pests and weeds, which makes it easier to manage. Nevertheless, if you're going to need a higher yield from your garden then you ought to find more space to grow your plants. This is where a garden plot on your yard will come into play. You just have to decide on convenience versus higher yield.

If you have some space on your yard then you can spare a small area to grow your herbs. However, more space means more work. You need to spend more time caring for the soil as well. Expect to do some of the itty gritty job since you will need to till the ground, remove weeds, and do a lot of trimming (some herbs tend to hog the open space leaving less room for other plants and herbs). Since you're going to grow your herbs in the open, you also have to deal with weeds and other pests. If you have a pet dog or cat then you should also provide some means of keeping them away from your precious medicinal herbs.

The actual location of your herb garden also matters, whether you're growing your herbs in your yard or in containers. Will the garden be located in a sunny spot? Figure out which herbs need more sun and place them where they can get the most sunlight. Is your window facing southwards? Then find out what medicinal herbs grow with less sun or will be better off in the shade.

The bottom line here is to be realistic with your expectations with regard to the space and location of your garden. The amount of space available and the garden's location will important factors to consider when you choose which medicinal herb to grow.

4. Work with Paper before You Work with Garden Spades

You don't want to go gung ho when you plant your home based herb garden. You may end up having too many plants than you have room for them. Now, here's a simple yet practical tip – plan your garden on paper.

The first step is to measure just how much space you have available. Use a ruler, tape measure, or better yet a measuring meter. Figure out how many square feet you have available for your herbs. If you're growing your herbs at the window sill then figure out how much space your herbs can occupy before they become a nuisance inside the house. Remember, some herbs tend to extend their branches and leaves while others may be able to reach high up to the ceiling.

Get the actual dimensions of the space you're going to work with. You don't need to make exact measurements down to the last centimeter. Now that you have a rough idea of the length and width of your gardening space, it's time to make your sketch. As a rule of thumb, you want to assign one square foot for each plant or herb. That way you're giving the roots enough room to spread and enough space for the branches to stretch out. If you end up with some extra space that doesn't square up to exactly one square foot then find some herbs that won't require that much space (e.g. herbs that tend to crawl upward on a pole).

If you're dealing with a huge garden plot and you can't figure out which herb should go into each square foot then don't be afraid to call on a designer. That can be anyone who has had a lot of experience with making and growing gardens. If you know a gardener or a landscape artist who has done that sort of work then ask for their opinion. Bring your pen and paper sketch to them and ask for suggestions. Their ideas may cost you a few bucks but those expert insights will be priceless in the long run.

5. Decide on How Many Herbs You Want to Grow and What Kind

If this is your first time to grow an herb garden from home then you better start small but plan big. You don't want to start working with 12 different kinds of herbs at once. You need to learn how each type of herb buds, grows, and behaves as the months go by (yes, months!). A good number to start will be 2 different herb species and a total of 4 or 5 plants. If you work with 2 types of herbs then get 2 plants for each herb. If one plant from each species dies then you at least have a 50% success rate for both types of herbs. Remember the rule – start small but plan your garden big time.

If you need some ideas on the types of medicinal herbs you can grow in your home garden then don't worry. We have a few suggestions in a later chapter of this book. Just remember that you will only need to start with a few plants if you're gardening at home for the first time.

If you have no idea which kind of herb will grow best in your area then you should ask local gardeners. Some herbs require more moisture than others while some herbs may not be suited to certain climates. Local gardeners will usually have a good idea what type of herb will grow given the conditions in your local area. Here's a small tip if you live in the colder parts of the country: plant your herbs on the windowsills during the colder months and then move the containers to an open lot during summer. That way you can have herbs lasting the whole year.

6. Watch Out for the Aggressive Herbs

Note that some herb plants are more aggressive than others. In fact, some herbs are actually invasive. These herbs tend to absorb all the nutrients from the soil or even grow faster than any other plant in your garden. Examples of these herbs include yarrow and peppermint.

In case you plan to grow your herbs on your yard, you should avoid planting these herbs directly into the soil of your yard. Best practice dictates that it is better for you to grow these overly aggressive herb species in containers so their reach will be limited. If you fail to keep them in check then you risk these herbs taking over your entire garden. Do yourself a favor; grow them in containers that are large enough for them to be happy.

7. Do I Do Seeds or Do I Do Starts?

This is a common question that comes up when people do any form of gardening for the first time. Beginners usually ask whether they should start growing plants using seeds or starts. Considering the cost, seeds are more practical simply because they are cheaper. However, growing your herbs from seeds may not be the best option if you're growing your herb garden for the first time. In case you're planning to grow your herbs from seeds you ought to know that you're risking the possibility that they may (or may not) grow beyond the first weeks after being planted. They are usually a bit fragile during such time.

8. Care for the Soil – Check for Drainage

We have already gone over fertilizers in the previous section. That's basically one way to care for the soil on your yard or the soil you will use in your container garden. Another important detail with regard to soil care is the amount of drainage. You see, even though water is a good thing for plants and herbs especially, too much water is a big problem for them. Your herbs will tend to get sickly and may eventually die if the soil is too moist.

If you're doing some container gardening for your herbs then make sure that there are enough holes at the bottom of your container for the excess water to seep out. Since you also don't want the soil to run through the holes it's also a great idea to fill the bottom with gravel first. That way, the water goes out faster and the soil is better retained inside the pot or container.

Most garden soils in your yard will drain off easily – unless of course you live in a swamp where there's no way for the water to drain. However, do take note that there are certain types of soil that still have poor drainage even if they are far away from bodies of water and marsh.

To check the drainage of the soil in your yard, here's what you can do. Grab a shovel and dig a hole in your yard where you plan to grow your garden. Dig a hole using a shovel (if you don't have one then use your garden spade) about a foot deep into the ground. Next, fill the hole with water. Wait until the soil absorbs all the water in the hole. After that, fill the hole with water again. This time wait for about an hour and then, using a ruler, measure how much water has been drained from the hole.

Now here's the deal, if after an hour the soil drains less than a couple of inches from the surface then the soil in your yard has poor drainage. If the water drained is more than two inches from the top then you have good drainage. In case you find out that the soil in your yard has poor drainage that means that the soil underneath it may have too much clay content. Clay holds water and keeps it from running off elsewhere. This means that more water is retained in your garden soil. Now, don't worry. There are ways to improve the drainage of your yard's garden soil. In fact we have an entire chapter dedicated to that. You can jump to it if you want to later on.

Chapter 2: Easy Guide to Successfully Grow Herbs and Medicinal Plants at Home

Follow this easy step-by-step guide to start with your medicinal herb garden at home:

1. Choose your herbs. When growing medicinal herbs at home, it is important to have a good variety of herbs as well as companion plants. Some of the good choice include the following:

   - Hot pepper

   - Strawberries

   - Oregano

   - Thyme

   - Lime basil

   - Mint

   - Common basil

   - Sage

   - Lemon balm

   - Sweet marjoram

2. Prepare your pot or garden plot if you want to grow your herbs in your yard. Be sure that the pots that you will be using for your medicinal plants have holes at the bottom to provide good drainage. With a grit or gravel, pour to about a quarter of the pot's depth. This will allow the water to steep out from the soil's bottom.

3. Fill. When the gravel is already in place, begin to fill the pot with soil-based or multi-purpose compost. Fill t about three (3) quarters of the pot's remaining space.

4. Begin planting – put the medicinal plants into the pot, with around 15 centimeters between each stem. Squeeze every plant lightly from its temporary pot. To encourage the plants to spread out, tease the roots from the root ball.

5. Put the trailing plants near the edge and the taller ones in the center of the display. This technique will endure the best growth for your plants. DO not worry if the display may seem to appear messy at first. This will begin to fill out and look lush in just a few weeks.

6. Fill in the spaces around the plants. When you are already satisfied with the positions, begin filling in the gaps in between the plants with compost. Tightly push the compost into the spaces by pushing your fingers deep into the soil. Be careful not to injure the roots. Add more if needed. To avoid overflowing when being waters, leave a few centimeters between the rim of the pot and the soil.

7. Top the plants. Cut the taller plants' top. This will encourage them to bush out and give more fresh leaves to pick during harvest time.

8. Fertilize regularly. Purchase a controlled release fertilizer which should last a whole season. This will mean that you won't have to feed the pot again.

9. Water. Water your plants thoroughly or until the water begins to drain out of the pot's bottom. Medicinal plants usually like to dry out between watering and some types of medicinal plants such as Rosemary can easily be over-watered.

The Beginners Guide to Medicinal Plants 2nd Edition

Growing herbs and medicinal plants at home is an easy yet a very rewarding hobby. Below are seven (7) key steps that will surely help you to successfully grow a healthy medicinal herb at home:

1. Keep an eye on Pests

   Medicinal herbs are generally not bothered so much about pests as much as flowers and vegetables can be. In an indoor garden however, the non-natural conditions may increase the possibility of a pest problem. To keep pests from damaging your medicinal plants in your indoor garden, make sure to keep a close eye. At the very first sight of infestation, make use of a soapy spray. You may also handpick any pests that you may have come to notices and put sticky traps to get rid of the rest.

2. Water your plants regularly

   Medicinal herbs require thorough attention when it comes to watering. Whether your medicinal plants like drier conditions or extra moisture, it is never a good idea to have plants to be sitting in water.

3. Apply fertilizer

   Always keep in mind that medicinal plants grown indoors require a special fertilization schedule than those which are planted in an outdoor environment.

4. Be mindful of the soil

   Indoor gardening soil needs to have effective exceptional drainage. It also needs to be light. Whether your medicinal plants like drier conditions or with extra moisture, having your plants to sit in water is never a good idea. Specifically buy potting soil. You may also prepare your own by using a part of peat moss, a part of sand and a part of bagged potting soil.

5. Ensure proper circulation

Medicinal plants require sufficient airflow to keep pests and bacterial organisms at bay. Just make sure to keep the air moving in the area where you will grow your medicinal plants.

6. Check your temperature

Keep your planting area at constant temperature. The ideal temperature for a home garden is about 60 to 70 degrees.

7. Provide enough light

Provide about 14 to 16 hours of artificial light to keep your medicinal plants healthy. You can also alternatively expose them to natural light for about 6 hours a day.

Chapter 3: The Best Medicinal Plants to Grow at Home

Do you have a small space at home to grow some plants? Why not grow some medicinal plants? Growing your own medicinal plants will not only get a lot of enjoyment but this will also provide medicinal relief in the comforts of your own home. While herbal remedies must never take the place of professional health care, it would be nice to have a sense of self-help should you ever end up having to need instant relief. Below is a list of the best plants to start your own personal medicinal plants garden:

1. Echinacea – this herb is also popularly known as the purple coneflower. Echinacea is an American perennial wildflower which is popularly known for its stimulating effects in the immune system. Preparations made with this wonder herb are used for the treatment of flu, colds, minor infections and a wide range of various illnesses.

2. Lavender – is medicinal plant which is commonly used as a fragrance these days. Lavender has been widely used since ancient times to reduce swelling, provide relief for rashes and itching and to treat burns, bug bites and other skin orders.

3. Lemon Balm – Prepare potent lemonade by adding bruised lemon balm leaves into your drink. This herb is commonly used as a calming "night tea" to combat insomnia. It can also make an effective topical relief for cold sores.

4. Comfrey – The roots of this wonder herb are cooked and mashed to make a potent topical relief for sprains,

burns, bruises and arthritis. Just do not eat it. There is a study which reported that this herb can potentially damage the liver in eaten in significant amounts.

5. St. John's Wort – this wonder herb can lift the mood very well that you must keep from using this when you are already taking other forms of anti-depressants. The flowers and leaves of this herb may be used to prepare a tea. They can also be soaked in liquor to make a tincture. In a recent announcement, the FDA warned the public that there was a risk of adverse reactions between this herb and certain prescription drugs used for the treatment of cancer, transplant rejection, heart disease and AIDS, among others.

6. Borage – this potent herb has beautiful flowers that may be soaked in alcohol to prepare a powerful tonic that can boost your mood. The flowers and leaves may be used in tea preparations, eaten raw or soaked in liquor or wine to flavor the drink. The fresh plant provides a salty flavor with a cucumber-like smell.

7. Peppermint – this medicinal plant can be an effective tonic to promote better digestion. However, peppermint and any other strong mints such as pennyroyal must not be taken by women who are pregnant or possibly be pregnant. Drinks and foods that have fresh strong mint leaf can be harmful to the baby.

8. Pennyroyal – just like peppermint, pennyroyal is a great smelling mint which can be crushed and topically applied to the skin as a very powerful insect repellent. The leaves of pennyroyal can be crushed and topically applied to wounds as an antiseptic agent. It can also be used in tea preparations to tame upset stomach, however, do not over do it. The maximum

recommendation is 2 cups daily. Consuming more than this recommendation may cause cramps and nausea.

9. Aloe vera – is a plant native to tropical Africa. This plant has spread worldwide as a first medicinal herb that provides soothing effects for scalds and burns. Aloe vera is best grown in a container so that it can be easily transferred indoors during the winter season.

10. Yarrow – for someone who's about to start a medicinal garden at home, yarrow is usually the top pick. This herb is a beautiful perennial plant that can serve a lot of different uses. Crushed yarrow flowers and leaves may be directly applied to scratches and cuts to reduce the chances of infections and to stop bleeding.

11. Slippery Elm – the inner back of this wonder herb can be ground and made into a nutrient-rich porridge-like soup. This can be an effective remedy for sore throat. In addition to this, the inner bark of this herb can be soothe irritations in the digestive tract.

12. Fenugreek – the seeds of this medicinal plant are nourishing and used to:

- Restore a dull sense of taste

- Freshen the breath

- Ease labor pains

- Ease painful menstruation

- Help in insufficient lactation

- Promote better digestion

- Help for late onset diabetes

- Darin off sweat ducts

- Treat inflammation and ulcers of the intestines and stomach

- Reduce blood cholesterol levels

- Inhibit cancer of the liver

- Encourage weight gain

13.   Feverfew – is a plant which can be made into tea for the treatment of fevers, colds and arthritis. This plant is said to have sedative properties. It can also regulate menstruation. A feverfew infusion may be used to bathe swollen feet. It can also be made into a tincture for the treatment of bruises. Chewing about 4 pieces of leaves daily has been proven to be an effective cure for some migraine headaches.

14.   Comfrey – an herb which contains allantoin. This substance is a cell proliferant which boosts the natural replacement of body cells. Comfrey is widely known for its ability to build strong teeth and bones in children. Comfrey is safer to use externally than internally. This wonder herb is used to treat a wider variety of health issues including the following:

- Varicose veins

- Eczema

- Sores

- Sprains

- Bruises

- Cuts

- Acne

- Severe burns

- Varicose and gastric ulcers

- Arthritis

- Sprains

- Broken bones

- Bronchial problems

15.   Milk Thistle – this powerful herb can protect and improve the function of the liver. This herb may be taken internally to help treat the following:

- The effects of a hangover

- The growth of cancer cells in prostate, cervical and breast cancer

- Insulin resistance in patients suffering from type 2 diabetes who also have cirrhosis

- Increased cholesterol levels

- Liver inflammation or hepatitis

- Jaundice

- Gall bladder diseases

- Liver diseases

16.   Wu Wei Zi – the fruit of this herb are reported to stimulate the central nervous system when used in low doses. In large doses, the fruits are said to depress the central nervous system while regulating the cardiovascular system. The seeds of this herb are used in the treatment of cancer. When used externally, this herb is used to treat allergic and irritating skin

problems. Internally, this herb is used to treat the following conditions:

- Diabetes
- Hepatitis
- Hyperacidity
- Poor memory
- Insomnia
- Palpitations
- Chronic diarrhea
- Involuntary ejaculation
- Urinary disorders
- Night sweats
- Asthma
- Dry coughs

17.   Sage – the latin name for this herb, "salvia", means to heal. When used internally, this herb treats the following conditions:

- Menopausal problems
- Femal sterility
- Depression
- Anxiety
- Excessive salivation
- Excessive perspiration

- Excessive lactation

- Liver issues

- Flatulence

- Indigestion

When used externally, sage is used for:

- Vaginal discharge

- Skin infections

- Gum infections

- Mouth infections

- Throat infection

- Skin infections

- Insect bites

18.   Turkey Rhubarb – this herb is popularly known for its beneficial and positive effect on the digestive system. Even children can take advantage of the beneficial effects of this herb because it is gentle enough. In low doses, the roots can serve as an astringent tonic for better digestion while higher doses may be used as laxatives. In addition to this, turkey rhubarb is also known to treat the following:

- Skin eruptions because of toxin accumulation

- Menstrual problems

- Hemorrhoids

- Gall bladder problems

- Liver diseases

- Diarrhea

- Chronic constipation

19.   Ginseng – is one of the most highly repudiated medicinal herbs in the orient. This wonder herb is touted for its ability to promote overall health, and general body vigor. The roots of this amazing medicinal plant is used to:

- Treat insomnia

- Address lack of appetite

- Treat debility related to old age

- Boost resistance against diseases

- Reduce levels of cholesterol

- Reduce blood sugar levels

- Enhance stamina

- Promote secretion of hormones

- Relax and stimulate the nervous system

20.   Evening Primrose - the young roots of this medicinal plant can be consumed like a vegetable. The shoots may also be eaten as a salad. The roots of this wonder herb can be applied to bruises and piles. The roots may also be made into tea for the treatment of bowel pains and obesity. However, the more valuable parts are the bark and the leaves which are made into evening primrose oil, which is popularly known to treat the following conditions:

- Alcohol-associated liver damage

- Rheumatoid arthritis

- Brittle nails

- Acne

- Eczema

- Hyperactivity

- Premenstrual tension

- Multiple sclerosis

21.　　Tea tree – even the aborigines have utilized the leaves of tea tree for medicinal purposes, such as chewing fresh leaves to ease headaches. The twigs, and leaves are made into tea tree oil which has antiseptic, antibacterial and antifungal properties. Tea tree oil definitely deserves a place in every household medicine cabinet. Tea tree oil is widely used for the treatment of the following illnesses:

- Minor burns

- Nits

- Cold sores

- Insect bites

- Warts

- Athlete's foot

- Acne

- Vaginal infections

- Thrush

- Chronic fatigue syndrome

- Glandular fever

- Cystitis

22. Great yellow gentian – the root of this powerful herb which is used to treat digestive problems. It is also capable of stimulating the digestive system, gallbladder and the liver. When taken internally, it is used to treat the following conditions:

- Anorexia

- Gastric infections

- Indigestion

- Liver complaints

Chapter 4: Ten (10) Most Common Herb and Medicinal Garden Mistakes and How to Avoid Them

Common Mistake No. 1: Not applying any fertilizers.

Once you have herbs and medicinal plants planted and growing, it is very essential to keep them growing healthy with the use of a light, all purpose fertilizer. Apply a compost tea once every week to give your herbal and medicinal plants a boost. Herbs and medicinal plants are going to be harvested a lot of times during the growing season. This only means that your plants will be need an extra boost in order to keep their growth cycle for an extended time. When applying fertilizer, make sure to keep the soil hydrated and not the leaves themselves along with the compost tea. This practice will be healthier for the plant and contaminations in the leaves will also be avoided.

Common Mistake No. 2: Not protecting the plants enough.

While the herbal and medicinal plants are known to be hardy and resistant to diseases and bug problems, they can still arise. A lot of times, herbal and medicinal plant gardeners are scared to employ any strategy to safeguard their plants. This should not be the case. There are a lot of homemade and organic controls that are safe to use for edible herbal and medicinal plants. Organic gardening begins before the plant is even in place. Good soil and beneficial insects work altogether towards a chemical free herbal and medicinal garden.

Common Mistake No. 3: Not watering the plants properly

The needs of herbal and medicinal plants are very minimal. While they are very easy to maintain and care for, these plants will be providing you with fresh harvest all season. Herbal and medicinal plants however require proper watering schedule in order to remain free from stress.

Herbal and medicinal plants should be watered in the early morning, if possible. In this way, the water will soak deeper into the soil without having to deal with any evaporation issue. Always keep the soil around the plant hydrated and never water over the leaves as this will only promote diseases and mildews. Good mulch is important for your herbs as well. This will keep the soil hydrated and may extend the time between watering. Avoid mulching right next to the plant's stem though as this may invite insects and other types of invaders to make their home.

Common Mistake No. 4: Not paying attention to the tiny details.

It is a must to watch herbal and medicinal gardens closely. You need to know what the plant should look like while it is healthy as this will allow you to immediately notice when a problem first happens. Keep an eye on any damaged stems, leaves and disturbed soil around the plant. If you notice that the stems and leaves are beginning to fade, turn brown or curl up, you will have became aware of the problem early enough to possibly save the plant.

Common Mistake No. 4: Spraying chemical compounds into the plants

Herbs and medicinal plants are usually rinsed and used fresh. They should never be exposed to any kind of treatment that may possibly be toxic or dangerous to those who would eat them.

Even if a product claims that it is safe to use around pets and people, you should look for the words safe for edibles. You cannot rinse a bunch of basil leaves with water and soup prior to using. There are a lot of ways to keep ahead of the problems that may require the application of chemicals. Weed on a regular basis, watch the plants closely for any insect infestation and use natural fertilizers such as compost tea.

Common Mistake No. 5: Allowing the flowers to turn into seeds.

Herbal and medicinal plants grow beautiful flowers. While a lot of these plants have edible flowers, it is not a great idea to allow the herb to flower early during the growing season. Once your plant flowers, this signals that its life cycle is about to come into an end. Your plant is growing a flower, then a seed, then it dies back for that particular season.

It is a better idea to keep any blossoms from forming in the first place. When you see a flower about to grow, just pinch the entire thing off. You will notice that the plant may become persistent. In such case, cut the entire stem or below the flower.

Common Mistake No. 6: overcrowding or planting incorrectly

It is common to purchase more plants that you can possibly grow in a given area. When purchasing your herbal and medicinal plants, read the plant tags that usually come with each pot. Keep an eye to the width and height of the fully grown plant. You can always grow a quick growing annual between the plants, if you do not prefer the look of mulch. It is always a good idea to underplant rather than plant the herbs too close to each other from the beginning. Over planting is a big waste for money as it will not allow your plants to grow a healthy root system. A sturdy root system will help them survive the winter and expand the next growing season.

Common Mistake No. 7: Not cutting back enough

Pruning is what makes a plant to grow fast and neat. Pruning an herb implies that you are actually harvesting the good tasting stems and leaves. If you omit pruning, the plant will only tend to grow taller on a few stems. The leaves will grow old, dry and fall off. This will result to longer stems without leaves, Pruning will also allow the plant to begin and finish its life cycle. By regular pruning, you are actually keeping the plant in its growing phase for as long as possible. It will keep the flowers from budding, promotes leaves and stems and keeps the plant producing for an extended period of time. Your plants will appear healthier and better, if pruned back on a regular basis.

Common Mistake No. 9: Growing the plants in the wrong environment.

Are you growing rosemary, a chalky and dry loving plant in a humid and moist area? Your plant will surely die off in about 2 weeks from wet feet. If you would like to grow plants in a shady area, go for plants that can tolerate less sun. The sun=loving plants will grow weak and pale from not enough bright sunlight daily. If you have neither too shady nor too sunny area, try planting in pots that can be rolled or moved to the optimal lighting conditions. It is not a matter of sufficient shading or sun but is just a matter of finding a way to be adaptable to what you already have.

Common Mistake No. 10: Choosing unhealthy medicinal and herbal plants

The very first chance you have to find the perfect plant is when you actually buy it. Search for healthy plants, bright in color, plenty of foliage and certainly not one egg or bug on it. Finding a single aphid means that there are a lot more that you cannot see, all awaiting for the perfect time to invade your other plants. Never have the sympathy for a weak looking plant, unless you have a lot of space to keep it isolated from your main garden area while you try to repair the damage. The effort and time to be spent in repairing an infested herb garden means wasted time. Take the extra step to look for the healthiest plants that you can purchase.

Chapter 5: Improving Your Yard's Drainage

Not all yards are the same and some yards drain water faster than others. There are two factors that make the difference from one yard to the other. These two factors are soil structure and soil texture. Understanding both will help you figure out why some soil drain easier than others. Let's deal with soil texture first.

When you talk about soil texture you're basically referring to just how much clay, silt, and sand is in your soil. There are different proportions of these soil elements in different areas. Having more clay in your garden soil will make it retain more water than the other materials. On the other hand, having more sand will make it lose more water. Unfortunately, there is very little you can do with regard to the constitution of your garden soil. The only thing you can do is to modify the soil structure – or basically how these soil materials are gathered together in your yard.

The following are tips you can use to change your yard's soil structure and improve its overall drainage.

Tip #1 – Add More Organic Material to Your Soil

The tilth of your garden soil can be improved by simply adding a layer of organic material over your plot (i.e. where you plan to plant your herbs). You can use compost to serve as the organic layer. You can make your own compost, which might take a while, or you can just buy it from a gardening store.

Adding compost to your soil will enlarge the pores on your garden soil. This in turn will improve the drainage. Since the pores tend to get bigger, then more water and air can go through the soil. You don't need a huge amount of compost to achieve this effect. You only need enough to make a layer that's a couple of inches thick on top of your garden plot. Once you have the plot covered with compost, use your garden spade to mix the old garden soil and compost. Make sure that the compost is well integrated into the soil.

Tip #2 – Enrich the Soil Using Cover Crops

This method will take a little more time compared to the results you will get in some of the other techniques mentioned here. However, this method not only improves your garden soil's drainage, it will also increase its quality. Using cover crops is actually the traditional way of improving any soil.

To get started with this traditional soil enrichment strategy, you will need some cover crops. Examples of these include clover as well as velch. You can get these from any garden supplier. The idea is to plant these cover crops on your garden plot. You will allow them to grow a bit but never reaching full maturity. Just grow them as much as you can but you will have to dig them back into the soil before the seeds start to set.

Cover crops tend to break the soil underneath using their roots. Doing so allows more water to pass through. The actual plant acts as some sort of green manure or green fertilizer, which improves the overall quality of the soil increasing its nutrient content when they are plowed back into the ground. As stated earlier, this method will take some time and it will definitely require more effort. However, the results are much better and longer lasting. These are factors you have to keep in mind when you make medicinal herb garden at home.

Tip #3 – Dealing with Hard Pan

Hard pans usually occur on your soil after some construction work. The soil gets too compressed thus allowing less water to pass through. This can happen after a house was constructed or after some home improvement was done on the property and a good deal of work was done outside (usually exactly on the soil where you want to grow herbs).

A hard pan is usually only a couple of feet deep, but they can be thicker too. The solution of course is to loosen up the soil a little bit. You can do that by digging a couple of feet into the soil. Remember to do your digging during the dry season. Digging through hard pan when the soil is too moist won't bring you the results you're looking for.

You have to dig into the soil twice to make sure that the soil is loosened up really well. After all that hard digging, water the soil and allow it all to settle. Once the loosened soil settles, you can move on to improving the soil's quality. Now, in case the hard pan is thicker than 2 feet then you will have to do some drilling, which means more hard labor. Of course, you can always hire someone to do the heavy lifting.

Tip #4 – The Magic of Gypsum

Some people think that adding more into the soil can improve drainage. If you go back to what was said earlier, it was aleady mentioned that there is very little you can do about soil texture. However, you can alter how the clay and sand are grouped or clumped together. To do that, you don't add sand but you add gympsum or otherwise known as calcium sulfate.

Gympsum has a unique effect on the clay mixed into your garden soil. Remember that all yard soil has some clay mixed in it. Dig into your garden soil and add gympsum. Mix them well and water the soil mixture. Allow the water to settle. Gypsum will make the clay particles in your soil to pull together more. This in turn will make make the soil develop micro pores that allow more water and air to pass through. Bottom line, it's not said that you need – you need gypsum (calcium sulfate) to create more pore development on your garden soil.

Tip #5 – Using a Dry Well

This next tip will require a lot more effort than usual. Dig a large hole that is around two or three feet deep. This hole or well should be located at the area where the soil has poor drainage. Fill the hole with rocks or broken up pieces of bricks. Pour water into the well using your garden hose. The water in your dry well will then seep through the surrounding soil underneath. This will eventually improve the drainage in your garden.

Tip #6 –French Drain It!

A French drain is basically what it says – it's a drain. It drains water away from your plot so the roots don't get soaked. To build a French drain, dig a trench along the length of your garden plot. Best practice dictates that you should make a gradual incline leading away from your plot. The incline should be around 1 to 3 inches. With that sort of incline, the water will drain faster.

The trench should be around 1 ½ feet in depth. Line the bottom of the trench with 3 inches of gravel. Place drain pipes on top of the gravel to collect water. After that, cover the drain pipes with more gravel until it levels with the top soil. When the water trickles from the plot, it will run through the top gravel and then to the drain pipes. The water will then flow downward and away from your garden plot and away from your herbs.

Chapter 6: Herb Gardening During Winter

Hardly anything grows during winter. Most crops won't survive the cold touch of Jack Frost when the snow covers the land. But that shouldn't stop you from enjoying fresh herbs during the coldest times of the year. The solution of course is to transfer your gardening from the yard to a cozy spot inside your home.

If you had a pretty huge garden plot then you should pick samples of every medicinal herb in your collection. You will then have to grow the younger plants in containers and harvest the mature ones before the first signs of frost comes in.

Indoor herb gardening is fast becoming a popular hobby nowadays. The idea of having fresh herbs during the winter is quite attractive. Imagine adding a fresh sprig to a hot stew on a winter morning. That would be a really welcome treat. In the case of medicinal herbs, the usual aches and pain (not to mention coughs and itches) don't go away when winter walks in. The herbs that people can use to cure everyday ills will definitely be just as useful at any season of the year.

Another good reason for growing herbs indoors during winter is that they make your decor look more, well, green. You can wake up to a lot of refreshing green accents inside the house. Some medicinal herbs even smell nice too.

Transitioning from Yard to Indoor Containers

If you started with container gardening, then you are already a step ahead when it comes to growing medicinal herbs indoors for the winter. You should have at least some experience with indoor plant maintenance, dealing with pests, and caring for diseased plants inside the house. However, if you're transitioning from herb gardening in the yard then you will have some serious work to do.

The timing of your transition is a key factor here. It's okay to be early when moving your medicinal herbs indoors. But making a late transition is rather problematic and if the early frost comes in way ahead of time then you should immediately rush into a panic mode to save your herbs.

So, timing your move is important, which means you have to pay attention to the weather forecast. You should begin your transition before the first frost during the fall season. During this time of the year, the cold chill will be mild and you will have enough time to acclimate your medicinal herbs to indoor living conditions.

You don't just pick up your herbs and bring them inside the house. That will be a bit traumatic for them. Herbs need time to get used to environmental changes. They're living organisms too you know. Once you have transferred your plants into pots (in case you grew them in your yard) then you should move them near a doorway, in your garage, or on an enclosure like a porch. They will have to stay there for about two or more weeks.

Remember, herbs grown in your yard are accustomed to lots of sun and plenty of room for their roots. They need to get acclimated to reduced sunlight and lesser legroom. Give them time and lots of care during this transition period. Make sure that these herbs stay in a bright and cool spot. It may not have as much sunlight as your yard but make sure they can get all the sunshine available.

After a couple of weeks or even more, your herbs should already be acclimated. You will notice that they should have recovered. Some herbs may stop growing a bit when transferred to a container and moved to a new location. You'll know they're acclimated when they start growing like they used to. Some herbs get used to their new living conditions fast while others may even take a full month to get acclimated.

Once your herbs have acclimated to their new surroundings it's time to move them indoors before winter strikes. As stated in one of our tips in a different chapter, you should place your medicinal herbs in that part of the house where there is abundant sunlight. They're typically near windows that face southwards. If you don't have any windows facing in that direction then look for windows that are facing either to the east or west. Remember to keep your herbs at or near windows but not too close. Any leaf that comes in direct contact with glass during winter can get a good nip from the frost outside.

Remember to keep your medicinal herbs away from heat sources like a fireplace or the heater. These plants need protection from both heat and dryness. Speaking of dryness, you should also water them regularly. Water helps to keep the dust away aside from the fact that they need water to grow. Remember that you should hold back a little on the watering come December all the way to the middle of January. Remember to cultivate the pot soil using a fork – watering will eventually compact any kind of potted soil.

Since we've already mentioned water and heat, you should also keep an eye on the prevailing indoor temperature. Most herbs prefer the usual day time temperatures, which usually range from 65 degrees Fahrenheit up to 70 degrees Fahrenheit. Those are the best temperatures for most herbs during the day. However, make sure that the temperature drops a little bit at night. You can reduce the temperature making it 10 degrees cooler. Some herbs can take temperatures ranging within the 50's. Keeping your indoor temperature within these levels at these times will sort of mimic the outdoor temperatures that your herbs have been used to while they were yet living in your yard.

Maintaining the Plant Life Equation

We have already covered a good deal about light and temperature when you grow your medicinal herbs during winter. Another important reminder about watering your herbs is to ensure that your pots or containers have good drainage. Well, you may have read drainage (and more drainage) a lot of times in this book but that point couldn't be stressed enough especially during the winter. Herbs like a good bath albeit regularly however, they don't have an inclination towards wet feet. Meaning, they don't love having their roots soaked. If you notice that your pot or container remaining too heavy for too long after you water your herbs then it means that your pots don't have proper drainage. You can add some potting soil, some sand, or even some vermiculite to improve the drainage quality of your soil. If the pots lack holes then poke a few additional holes.

The type of pot you're using will also be a factor when judging drainage. Herbs grown in clay pots will definitely need a bit more water since clay pots usually drain well (sometimes too well). If the clay pot is at a window that's facing southwards then the herb will require more water. If you're using plastic containers or plastic pots then the herbs will require a little less water. If the plastic pot is at a window that's facing either east or west then it will require even less water.

Usual Problems You Can Experience During Winter

You might notice that your medicinal herbs will get a bit spindly when you grow them indoors for the winter. Don't worry about. That's a usual occurrence when you move any plant from the yard and into the house. The best living conditions for any type of foliage is outdoors – no doubt about it. Well, the good news is that once winter is over you can start moving your medicinal herbs back on your yard.

Even though spindly growth isn't something to worry about, you still should check your herbs regularly for the usual pests and other problems that they can have during winter. Any indoor herb, medicinal or culinary, will be prone to aphid damage, spider mites, and whitefly, since they will be in a rather weakened state. The solution of course is to provide them with the best living conditions possible (i.e. all the stuff we have mentioned here in this book).

In case you find a plant that has insects on it then make sure to isolate that plant. Keep it away from the other herbs and put it in quarantine. You can use soap sprays if you have an insect infestation. However, don't use it on seedlings. You should also remember that your soap spray should hit the insects to achieve the desired effect (i.e. killing them on contact). Of course the soap will come in contact with the plant so you have to wash them off. You should conduct your soap spraying treatment at night. You risk drying the leaves of your herbs if you spray them during the day time.

Additional Tips for Growing Medicinal Herbs During Winter

Just like any living organism, medicinal herb plants also need a good vitamin boost. Watering them is good but sometimes that isn't good enough especially if you really want to keep them healthy throughout the winter. You can add liquid seaweed as well as B1 plant mix to the water for your herbs. They contain essential vitamins, growth hormones, root hormones, and other necessary nutrients.

Note that any herb can drain the nutrients in a pot in just 10 days. That's how fast their roots can mine the nutrients from the soil especially if they're stuck inside a confined space such as a pot or container. You should stock up on nutrient mixes from the store. There are mixes that you can add to the soil and there are mixes that you can add to water.

You should also make sure to harvest your herbs when they are ready. Occassional trimming and harvesting from your medicinal herbs may be needed from time to time during winter. Doing so will keep your plants healthy. Depending on the type of herb you're growing, expect that you will need to do some harvesting from 4 up to 6 weeks since you moved your herbs indoors.

Chapter 7: Growing Medicinal Herbs for Profit

Other than growing medicinal plants as a hobby, some people have learned how profitable these herbs can be. There are people who have become keenly aware of the demand for herbs both medicinal and culinary. Of course, we'll only deal with the medicinal herbs in this book. Starting your very own herb business will include all the stuff we've discussed so far. That includes raising herbs, harvesting them, saving their seed, and selling your herbs.

There is already a market for herbs for big businesses, which basically include large pharmaceutical companies who are rushing to zero-in on the beneficial components of every medicinal herb on the planet. Well, their purpose is to create some brand new medicine from the plant components. However, there is also a growing market for medicinal herbs that is currently being served by small and medium enterprises. If you've found a knack for growing medicinal herbs and you think you want to make money out of this new hobby then by all means, read on.

A Few Examples of Successful Medicinal Herb Entrepreneurs

Note that you're not the first one to market medicinal herbs. There have been others before you and some have become quite successful. The story seems to repeat itself from one case to the other: a certain someone needed something to treat an ailment, finds an herb that cures, grows the herb for personal consumption, raises more herbs, sells it, and then makes good money. Well, some stories vary a little but they eventually end up in the same way – making good money out of a hobby. Examples of such peopple include Patricia

Winters (grows 15 acres of herbs today), Hariet Widmer (owner of Cherry Hill Herbs), and Roy E. Anderson (biggest chive grower in the country).

Is There Money to Be Made?

Back in 2013 a study was conducted by North Carolina University's Horticultural Science Department. The focus of the study was to answer the question of whether farmers can make a profit from growing medicinal herbs or not. The final answer was yes but of course, there were certain obstacles that were found. Of course, every new endeavor or enterprise will have obstacles. All types of businesses will have to take certain risks.

Back in 2011, nutritional product sales went up to 126 billion dollars. That represents a growth of higher than eigh percent. According to experts that they expect that sales for these products will grow about one percent or more each year since. And where do you think will manufacturers get their supplies to make their nutirional products? They'll get it from local medicinal herb farmers of course.

Raw material ingredients sales that require medicinal herbs grew to 11.3 billion dollars back in 2011. The figures today still show a persistent steady growth. This increase in sales is driven by the fact that manufacturers are concerned about increasing shipping costs from important their materials from abroad. They are also concerned about raw material contamination from overseas sources. So, if they can't get their raw materials (which includes herbs and such) overseas then they will purchase them from local manufacturers. Part of the push for buying local products is the rising support from local consumers. More consumers in the country today want to make sure that they're using products that contain organic materials. There's a growing demand for medicinal herbs and that demand will be filled by local farmers one way or another.

Understanding the Cost

Of course, raising your commercial herb garden from the ground up will entail some costs. To give you some sort of an idea, here are some figures of the costs of raising medicinal herbs in a garden the size of a 1/10th acre land:

- Planting Stocks (includes seeds and roots) will cost about $1,500 a year.
- Compost, fertilizer, etc. will cost $150 a year on average.
- Utilities and equipment costs will be at $700 a year.
- Certification costs will be at $100 a year.
- Packaging costs will be at $200 per year.

That's about $2,650 a year for your operating expenses. You don't have to cough up that entire amount on the first month. Well, at least you already have an idea just how much you'll have to spend in a year.

Some Common Pitfalls That You Should Avoid

Some farmers, of course, failed to make profit at certain times. Some even gave up on the idea of selling medicinal herbs. Remember that selling these kinds of herbs is not the same as selling herbs on the market. There is a different approach for farmers and small growers. Here are some pitfalls that ought to avoid:

- Not consulting a buyer before planting an herb: Herb farmers and homegrown medicinal herb growers should first consult buyers before they start growing herbs. They should agree on the type of herb, size, quantity, and packaging. Once farmers and producers know the standards set by buyers then they can start growing, harvesting, packing, and then selling the herbs to a ready buyer. If you don't abide by the buyer's expectations then don't expect them to buy your goods.

- Not processing herbs according to specifications: Note that different buyers have different specifications. Some buyers prefer fresh herbs. Some buyers only want the seeds of herbs. Some buyers want herb roots or leaves sun dried. There are buyers who want you to package your herbs in a certain way to make it easier for them to incorporate your products into their production system. There are all sorts of specifications and the main idea is to go with the buyer whose specs you can support. If a certain process or specification will entail too much cost or a cost that you can't shoulder then you ought to find another buyer.

- Not following GAPs: All buyers will only buy from medicinal herb producers who follow good agricultural practices (GAPs). Some even specify certain GAPs that should be followed. Sometimes they will even do a site inspection of your production facilities (aka your little farm) just to make sure you are up to standard. Learn these GAPs and abide by them. Some of them even help to keep the environment clean.

- Do you have the proper equipment: Some buyers want to get their supplies only from local herb producers who use the proper equipment. Learn what the current industry standard equipment is and use them. They may entail some additional costs but the profits that you can make because of them will pay for it in the long run. You can also expect a more efficient production if you use standard equipment.

Don't be dismayed if one buyer turns you down. Remember that there are many manufacturers who do buy medicinal herbs directly from farmers and small scale producers. Some of them even pay a small premium to local growers. There will always be someone who will want to buy your herbs. Just keep looking and avoid the above mentioned pitfalls.

Where Else to Find Buyers

Are there direct markets that you can try? The answer is yes. Other than the regular buyers (e.g. pharmaceutial companiens and manufacturers of health products) there are herbalism schools that will buy directly from farmers. If you have a county fair or festival then you can market your produce there as well. There are farmer's markets that allow herb farmers and small scale growers to display and sell their goods. Some healthy living practitioners will buy their supplies from local producers as well.

Nowadays you can also use the Internet as a resource to find buyers of your medicinal herbs. You can go to the American Herbal Products Association website and look for buyers, raw material suppliers, dealers, and just about anyone who would want to buy medicinal herbs.

Good Agricultural Practices

Now, we have mentioned GAPs earlier. Everyone is expected to follow these agricultural practices. As stated earlier, some buyers will even require their suppliers and farmers to follow additional practices before they buy your herbs. The following are some of the more common GAPs that you should know about:

- All herbs must be properly identified
- All herbs must be free from contaminants
- Specifications set by buyers and growers should be met
- Abide by all local agricultural laws
- Have good environmental stewardship
- Grower must practice good post harvest storage and harvest

- Harvests should be done during the most optimal time

As you can see, GAPs are not unreasonable. In fact, they are there only to ensure that only quality products reach the market.

The Matter of Production Records and All Sorts of Records

One of the big differences between growing medicinal herbs as a hobby and growing them for profit is record keeping. You will barely keep track of your production when you're growing herbs for your own consumption, right?All you want to do is to plant it, grow it, and use the herbs when the sniffles or aches come along. Since some medicinal herbs are also good for food then you may on occasion add them to your favorite stew.

But things are different when you do larger scale production and hope to make profit from your hobby. You will have to keep track of a lot of things. One important record you need to make is your site history. You should record what herbs have you grown and which ones you were successful at.

You should also keep track of your seed sources. You can't keep depending on seeds and starts suppliers. You should be able to successfully make your own seeds and starts. You should also record what sorts of products and manufacturing processes you have applied during your production efforts. You should also keep a record of when you planted certain herbs and when you harvested them. In case you have a buyer who wants dried herbs then you should also record the drying temperatures so that you already know how to properly process your buyer's orders next time around.

That's a lot of things to keep track of and you haven't even begun to record how much profit you have made in the last 3 to 5 years. If you want to grow medicinal herbs for profit you ought to do it for the long term. That means working on your business for about three to five years. That's your time frame for success. If you can make profit within that range then you can run this sort of business and make huge amounts of profits from what was just once your hobby—growing medicinal herbs in your backyard.

Chapter 8: Best Medicinal Herbs for Commerce

We have already provided a list of great herbs that you can grow on your backyard. The list below is something like that. It has some of the best selling herbs that you can grow and sell to potential buyers. The herbs are listed in no particular order. The demand for these herbs will shift at different times of the year. You should also note that this list is not comprehensive. There are other medicinal herbs that also have a pretty high demand. You should do your own market research and find out which herbs currently have a pretty good demand that you can supply locally.

Chamomile

Chamomile helps with a lot of digestive problems. Some people use it to get some good night sleep. You just have to make it into some sort of tea. The most profitable type of Chamomile is the German variant. Yes, there are other variants but many buyers want the German one. Of course, there is also a chance that you can find buyers who would want to buy other Chamomile variants as well so you should also look into that market.

St. John's Wort

We have already discussed St. John's Wort in the previous list of medicinal herbs. It provides immune support, it's great for colds, and helps with your mood. Most buyers want St. John's Wort supplies to reach full maturity. If you harvest them too early then you risk not being able to sell them to your intended buyer.

Lemon Verbena

This herb also helps with digestion issues. It also helps people sleep better. Many buyers will want only softwood stem cuttings. There are also buyers who will order fresh leaves. Make sure to follow your buyer's specifications with this herb.

Catnip

We all know that catnip is some sort of stimulant for cats. However, this herb is actually a sedative for human beings. It is usually used to produce products for stress as well as pain relief. Catnip is very easy to sell. In fact, this is one of the medicinal herbs that you can readily sell in local fairs, fund raisers, festivals, and even church sponsored events.

Marsh Mallow

When harvested fresh this medicinal herb works great for cough. When processed, then it can also be used to make products that treat a variety of skin conditions.

Lavender

Lavender doesn't only smell good, it also has a lot of meidicinal qualities as well. Some people call this herb as some kind of Swiss Army Knife of all the many different herbs on the planet since it has a lot of medicinal uses. Needless to say, there is a huge demand for lavender in the market.

Calendula

This herb is used for skin preparations and is useful for digestive problems. This is also one of the herbs that are very easy to grow in any garden in any part of the world.

Conclusion

Thank you again for purchasing this book!

I hope this book was able to help you to know how to successfully grow medicinal plants and herbs at home.

The next step is to follow the step-by-step guide and see your plants grow healthier each day.

Finally, if you enjoyed this book, please take the time to share your thoughts and post a review on Amazon. We do our best to reach out to readers and provide the best value we can. Your positive review will help us achieve that. It'd be greatly appreciated!

Thank you and good luck!

Check Out My Other Books

Below you'll find some of my other popular books that are popular on Amazon and Kindle as well. Simply click on the links below to check them out. Alternatively, you can visit my author page on Amazon to see other work done by me.

Coconut Oil for Easy Weight Loss

http://amzn.to/1i5f45p

Essential Oils & Aromatherapy

http://amzn.to/1ouuZTx

Superfoods that Kickstart Your Weight Loss

http://amzn.to/1eyHdku

The Best Secrets Of Natural Remedies

http://amzn.to/1gmHd7y

The Hypothyroidism Handbook

http://amzn.to/1emWfyR

The Hyperthyroidism Handbook

http://amzn.to/1kqLQCp

Essential Oils & Weight Loss For Beginners

http://amzn.to/Q83bFp

Top Essential Oil Recipes

http://amzn.to/1lSrhSC

Soap Making For Beginners

http://amzn.to/1fkmYwr

Body Butters For Beginners

http://amzn.to/1fWjwJe

Homemade Body Scrubs & Masks For Beginners

http://amzn.to/1jjLRIO

Carrier Oils For Beginners

http://amzn.to/1sbqUQP

Natural Homemade Cleaning Recipes For Beginners

http://amzn.to/1izDB2m

The Beginners Guide To Medicinal Plants

http://amzn.to/1vSujr6

The Beginners Guide To Making Your Own Essential Oils

http://amzn.to/1piUNSB

The Beginners Alkaline Miracle Diet

http://amzn.to/1sDVaVE

Thyroid Diet

http://amzn.to/1piW2RY

Essential Oils Box Set #1 (Weight Loss + Essential Oil Recipes

http://amzn.to/1qlYWWP

Essential Oils Box Set #2 (Weight Loss + Essential Oil & Aromatherapy

http://amzn.to/1qlYWWP

Essential Oils Box Set #3 Coconut Oil + Apple Cider Vinegar

http://amzn.to/1oIFZJw

Essential Oils Box Set #4 Body Butters & Top Essential Oil Recipes http://amzn.to/1jSxURJ

Essential Oils Box Set #5 Soap Making & Homemade Body Scrubs

http://amzn.to/RAvJYo

Essential Oils Box Set #6 Body Butters & Body Scrubs

http://amzn.to/RAvSel

Essential Oils Box Set #7 Top Essential Oils & Best Kept Secrets Of Natural Remedies

http://amzn.to/1gvsRCq

Essential Oils Box Set #8 Homemade Cleaning Recipes & Essential Oil Recipes

http://amzn.to/1gxFAVb

Essential Oils Box Set #9 Essential Oil and Weight Loss & Carrier Oils

http://amzn.to/1jmcEPP

Essential Oils Box Set #10 Hyperthyroidism Manual & Hypothyroidism Manual

http://amzn.to/1nHgJU4

Essential Oils Box Set #11 Carrier Oils for Beginners & Coconut Oil for Easy Weight Loss

http://amzn.to/1nHfy6X

Essential Oils Box Set #12 Essential Oils Weight Loss & Essential Oils Aromatherapy & Natural Homemade Cleaning Supplies & Top Essential Oil Recipes & Carrier Oils
http://amzn.to/1nHfy6X

Essential Oils Box Set #13 Superfoods & Essential Weight Loss & Essential Aromatherapy & Body Butters & Soap Making
http://amzn.to/1nUds6v

Essential Oils Box Set #14 Weight Loss & Apple Cider Vinegar & Body Butters & Homemade Body Scrubs & Coconut Oil for Beginners
http://amzn.to/1i1qYOd

If the links do not work, for whatever reason, you can simply search for these titles on the Amazon website to find them.

www.ingramcontent.com/pod-product-compliance
Lightning Source LLC
Chambersburg PA
CBHW071125280526
45787CB00003B/1178